YMCA Youth Fitness Test Manual

B. Don Franks, PhD

Professor and Director of
School of Health,
Physical Education,
Recreation, and Dance
Louisiana State University

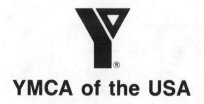

YMCA of the USA

Library of Congress Cataloging-in-Publication Data

Franks, B. Don.
   YMCA youth fitness test manual / by B. Don Franks.
     p.   cm.
   Bibliography: p.
   ISBN 0-87322-263-6
   1. Physical fitness--Testing--Handbooks, manuals, etc.   I. YMCA
of the USA. II. Title.
GV436.F72   1989
613.7'043--dc20   89-33612
                                              CIP

ISBN: 0-87322-263-6

Published for the YMCA of the USA by Human Kinetics Publishers, Inc.

Printed in the United States of America

10 9 8 7 6 5 4 3 2

Copies of this book may be purchased from the YMCA Program Store, Box 5077, Champaign, IL 61825-5077, (217) 351-5077

Contents

□

Preface

Physical fitness has been a common thread running through many YMCA programs for all ages. The YMCA's recent major program emphasis on youth health and fitness has resulted in a book on physical fitness *activities* (Thomas, Lee, & Thomas, in press) and in this book, providing a specific physical fitness *test* for children and youth. The Youth Fitness Test can be used with a special fitness unit or as part of other courses that have physical fitness as a goal.

Testing of physical fitness, health, and performance has a somewhat confusing history. Early "fitness" tests included muscular performance items and were used to try to predict both an individual's health and the ability to perform. Testing has since evolved into measures with three basic aims: (1) to diagnose disease; (2) to predict performance, or the ability to do specific work or athletic tasks; and (3) to evaluate positive health status (physical fitness).

An example of disease diagnosis is the interpretation of the electrocardiogram during a graded exercise test, utilizing the expertise of both cardiologists and exercise physiologists. The prediction of performance is becoming very specific and specialized (e.g., testing to determine who can be a successful fire fighter or an Olympic wrestler); it involves measurement specialists and coaches or employers. Testing for physical fitness helps evaluate current health status for persons of all ages. It may take the form of laboratory tests in a research center or field tests in a volunteer agency, school, or community fitness program.

The YMCA Youth Fitness Test described in this booklet is a field test for the physical fitness of children and youth. Chapter 1, "What Is Physical Fitness?" defines physical fitness and its components and explains how fitness relates to an individual's present and future health. In the second chapter, "The YMCA Youth Fitness Test," the test is described. Test validity and techniques for more accurate measurement precede the practical instructions for test administration, which are written in easily understood language. Chapter 3, "Application of Test Results to Fitness Programming," suggests three criteria for providing recognition to participants: exhibiting fitness behavior, meeting fitness standards, and accomplishing specific fitness goals; the latter two involving test scores. Use of test scores in program development also is briefly reviewed.

The test procedures and measurement standards are based on the best current thinking of exercise and measurement specialists. In addition, an early version of the test was field-tested by several YMCAs, and test procedures were modified on the basis of Y directors' feedback. As with any test, periodic revisions will be desirable as research provides information for better testing procedures and fitness standards.

B. Don Franks
April 1989

Acknowledgments

Thanks to the YMCA for being in the forefront of physical fitness over the years. The leadership, programs, and materials that the Y has provided have made a contribution to fitness. I also appreciate the feedback I received from the many YMCA directors who used an earlier version of this test:

Kathy DePatta
Las Vegas YMCA
Las Vegas, NV

David Engelhardt
Decatur County YMCA
Greensburg, IN

Roberta Kelzer
Monroe County YMCA
Bloomington, IN

Julee Lefebure
Cass County Family YMCA
Logansport, IN

Lyn Schlegel
Central YMCA
Fort Wayne, IN

Lynne Vaughan
Battle Creek Y Center
Battle Creek, MI

Paul Versnik
South Lexington YMCA
Lexington, KY

Ted Weigel
Arthur Jordan Branch YMCA
Indianapolis, IN

Ralph Wheeler
Pikes Peak YMCA
Colorado Springs, CO

I am indebted to Ed Howley and others with whom I have coauthored books and articles about fitness. They have helped me form and refine my concepts concerning fitness and fitness testing. They may recognize some of the material!

In a more general way, I am indebted to my students and professional colleagues, too numerous to list, who have educated me over the past three decades. Many measurement and fitness specialists with whom I have worked are now providing the leadership for fitness testing and position statements for the Institute of Aerobics Research; the American College of Sports Medicine; the American Alliance for Health, Physical Education, Recreation and Dance; and other groups. A special thanks to my former advisors, George Moore and T.K. Cureton, Jr., who sparked my interest in evaluation and fitness.

CHAPTER 1

What Is Physical Fitness?

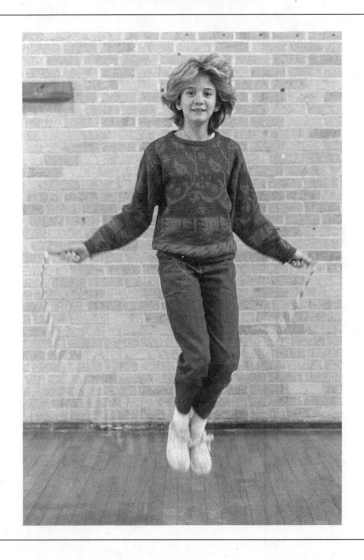

□

The term *physical fitness* means many things to many people. For some, it means physical activities— anything from archery to weight lifting. For others, it means getting your weight down, or having a healthy cardiovascular system. Thus, it is not surprising that physical fitness *tests* include many different characteristics and performance tasks.

To understand what *physical* fitness is, it's first necessary to know what *fitness* itself is. *Fitness* is one's capacity to achieve the optimal quality of life. It is an ever-changing, many-faceted state that includes healthy mental, social, spiritual, and physical behaviors. Fitness is based on good health, and it includes individual physical performance goals. The fit person possesses all of the following:

- Cardiorespiratory endurance
- Mental alertness
- Meaningful relationships with others
- Desirable level of fat
- Desirable level of strength
- Desirable level of flexibility
- A healthy low back

Being fit means being able to enjoy life fully, with a low risk of developing major health problems. Figure 1.1 shows a continuum of fitness states from death to life. The person who is most fit will be closest to life. Any changes in fitness characteristics can move an individual from one place to another on the continuum.

Although no single definition of physical fitness is used by everyone, there is a wide consensus that the primary physical fitness concept is *a relationship to positive health.* This concept is increasingly being endorsed by exercise and measurement specialists and by professional groups such as the American Alliance for Health, Physical Education, Recreation and Dance (1988); the American College of Sports Medicine (1988); and the American Heart Association (1986). The concept fits well with the YMCA's long-standing commitment to health-related physical fitness.

3

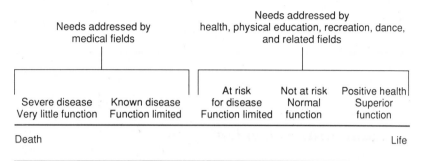

Figure 1.1. Fitness continuum.

Goals of Positive Health

We can think of positive health as having a number of goals, which are ordered in layers (see Table 1.1). Some of these layers—lack of disease, fundamental movement, and physical fitness—are general concerns for everyone. The others—energy for everyday tasks and performance—must be individualized for each person's lifestyle.

Table 1.1   Goals of Positive Health

Positive health goal	Sphere of concern
Lack of disease	General
Fundamental movement	General
Energy for everyday tasks	Individual
Physical fitness	General
Performance	Individual

Lack of Disease

The first layer is the medical diagnosis of freedom from disease. Medical, health, and fitness leaders work to prevent illness. Although the incidence of many childhood diseases has been greatly reduced, children and youth still need to learn to identify signs, symptoms, and test scores that might indicate possible medical problems. Freedom from disease is an important first step, but, as terms such as "wellness" indicate, there is much more to health and fitness than being without disease.

Fundamental Movement

The second layer of positive health is the ability to perform physical movements common in everyday life—walking, running, throwing, catching, jumping. Being able to perform these movements at levels appropriate for age and development is important for children.

Physical education programs for children emphasize fundamental movement experiences in dance, exercise, games, and gymnastics. Some people question whether children's physical education should stress creative movement in dance, games, and gymnastics or should stress fitness. This is a useless argument: Physical education should do both! The YMCA youth fitness program has a good balance of both fundamental movement activities and fitness activities.

Energy for Everyday Tasks

The ability to carry out daily activities without undue fatigue is the third layer. The amount of energy needed to achieve this goal will differ depending on the individual child's family, school, and leisure activities. Having the energy to do physical tasks is the primary concern of this layer.

Physical Fitness

The next positive health layer is physical fitness, the state of physical well-being that is related to optimal health. That state consists of having sufficient levels of the components of physical fitness (to be discussed) that contribute to developing and maintaining good health.

Performance

This final layer relates to participation in sport or other physical tasks. Performance is the development of skills and abilities needed to do a selected activity well enough to compete with others (or oneself) at a desired level. This level varies among individuals: Some will be happy to finish a 5K run in less than 30 minutes; others may want to play in the "A" division of the youth soccer league. The specific skills and abilities to be developed, such as agility, balance, coordination, power, or speed, also vary with the activity.

Components of Physical Fitness

The YMCA Youth Fitness Test identifies physical fitness in terms of five components:

- Cardiorespiratory endurance
- Relative leanness
- Healthy low back function
- Muscular strength and endurance
- Flexibility

These components meet the basic fitness standard of a relationship with positive health; they also are components that can be improved in a good fitness program such as the YMCA youth fitness program. In addition, each component has a valid field test.

Cardiorespiratory Endurance

Cardiorespiratory endurance (CRE) is also called cardiovascular or aerobic capacity. It includes the ability of the heart, lungs, and blood vessels to get oxygen to the muscles and the ability of the muscle fibers to use that oxygen to obtain the energy needed for physical activity. CRE meets the criteria for a fitness component because increased CRE is related to a higher quality of life and low levels of CRE cause greater health risks. CRE can be improved in people of all ages through aerobic activities.

Relative Leanness

The human body is composed of muscle, bone, organs, and fat, the total of which makes up body weight. From a fitness perspective, body weight is divided into fat weight and lean (non-fat) weight. Fat weight includes fat that is necessary for survival, called *essential fat,* and all extra fat. Lean weight includes all tissues and organs other than fat. For example, a child whose body is 30% fat and who weighs 70 pounds is carrying 21 pounds of fat weight (30% of 70 pounds) and 49 pounds of lean weight (70 – 21).

Essential fat averages 3% of body weight for all children and for men, and 12% of body weight for women after puberty. The higher value for women reflects the fact that fat is deposited in the breasts and hips at puberty.

Essential fat sets the lower healthy limit of body fatness. Too little fat can cause severe health problems. A small amount of extra fat (about 10% to 15%) above the essential fat can be tolerated without health problems. Too much fat, however, can lead to serious psychological and physical health problems (such as heart disease).

The proportion of fat on the body, or relative leanness, meets the criteria for a fitness component in that too little or too much fat can increase the risk of serious health problems, while an optimal amount is related to positive health. A fitness program that includes exercise and good nutrition can help people achieve healthy levels of fat.

Healthy Low Back Function

Low back pain is responsible for much avoidable suffering. The incidence of low back pain in the United States has increased over the past several decades and is related to the sedentary lifestyle many have adopted. Many factors can cause low back pain, such as the following:

- Structural abnormalities
- Disease
- Accidents
- Improper lifting of heavy objects
- Poor posture
- Lack of warm-up before vigorous activity

- Lack of abdominal strength or endurance
- Lack of flexibility in the back and legs
- Inability to cope with stress

Being free from back pain is certainly one aspect of a healthy life. A fitness program that includes both exercises for flexibility and muscular strength and endurance in the midtrunk area and education on how to prevent back injury can improve this fitness component for most individuals.

Muscular Strength and Endurance

A certain amount of muscular strength and endurance is needed to perform numerous daily tasks. Although high-level sports performers such as varsity athletes need separate tests and training for muscular strength and muscular endurance, most people who are interested in fitness can combine the two.

Abdominal strength and endurance are important to the prevention and relief of low back pain. Strength and endurance in other parts of the body are essential for daily life. In addition, activities that improve muscular strength and endurance may help maintain desirable levels of bone density, thus helping to prevent osteoporosis in later life. Muscular strength and endurance can be increased with fitness program activities that overload the muscles.

Flexibility

The ability of a joint to move through a normal range of motion is called *flexibility*. When joints are flexible, everyday tasks can be completed without undue strain. A lack of flexibility can be related to health problems, with low back pain being one example. Static stretching, which is a part of the warm-up and cool-down in most fitness programs, can improve flexibility.

Now that all the components of the test are identified, chapter 2 presents the testing procedures for each.

CHAPTER 2

The YMCA Youth Fitness Test

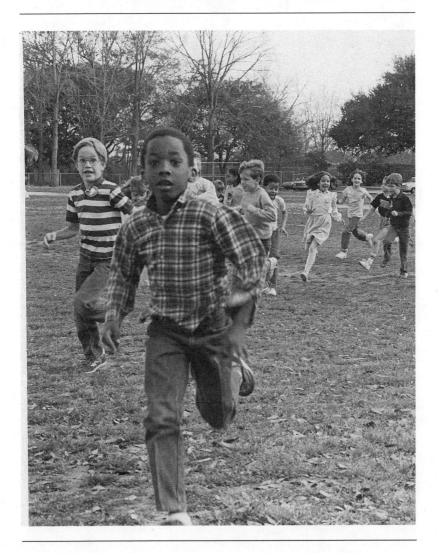

□

This chapter supplies all the information necessary for administering the YMCA Youth Fitness Test, which is actually a battery of five test items. The test items measure the five physical fitness components as shown in Table 2.1.

Table 2.1   YMCA Youth Fitness Test Items

Fitness component	Test items
Cardiorespiratory endurance	One-mile run
Relative leanness	Triceps and calf skinfold measurement
Flexibility/healthy low back	Sit-and-reach test
Muscular strength/endurance	
Abdominal/healthy low back	Curl-ups
Arms	Modified pull-ups

Equipment and settings are described, along with instructions for testing. But before the Youth Fitness Test is described, information on its validity and on techniques for making testing more accurate is presented.

Test Validity

The most important question to raise about any test is "Does it measure the characteristic I'm interested in evaluating?" In other words, is the test *valid*? The first requirement for validity is *consistency*. Consistency includes the *reliability* of the test and the *objectivity* of the scores assigned by the testers. For a test to be reliable, it must provide the same score for the same person if the test is repeated (provided the fitness of the person has not changed). For objectivity to be shown, the test must give the same results regardless of who administers or scores it. An unreliable or nonobjective test cannot be valid.

After the consistency of a test is assured, there are three major ways to determine whether the test measures what it is supposed to: content, concurrent, and construct validity. *Content validity* means that the test seems to be a good one, based on logic, expert testimony, and widespread use. *Concurrent validity* means that the test provides information similar to that generated by one or more accepted tests of the same characteristic. *Construct validity* means that the test results reflect the theoretical understanding of the characteristic being tested.

Each of the fitness test items in the YMCA Youth Fitness Test has been shown to be reliable and objective when carefully administered by a trained professional. All test items have content validity. Fitness experts have recommended these tests, which have been used in numerous fitness programs and research projects to measure the selected fitness components.

An endurance run is the most practical field test for cardiorespiratory endurance. Runs of less than a mile involve more sprinting ability (which uses anaerobic metabolism) and thus are less related to aerobic capacity. Runs of more than a mile are good for conditioning, but they do not provide any more information about a person's CRE than a one-mile run. Timed runs, such as running as far as possible in 9 minutes, are also good CRE tests, but most practitioners prefer a running test for a set distance.

Measurement of body skinfolds is the best field method for estimating percent body fat (or fat weight, as described in chapter 1). A combination of triceps measurement with either subscapular or calf measurement has been shown to be the best predictor of percent fat for children and youth. Triceps and calf skinfold measurements are recommended because the calf is easier to measure than the subscapular region; the child's shirt does not need to be lifted to take the measurement.

The sit-and-reach test is the best field test for flexibility related to low back function. The use of a box to stabilize the feet gives more accurate measurements than the V-sit, which is the same movement done on the floor with lines marked for the feet. Some practitioners suggest testing each leg separately, as each leg is stretched separately during stretching exercises, but there doesn't appear to be enough additional information gained to make it worth taking the extra time.

Many fitness tests include a timed sit-up, with feet held, for abdominal endurance. However, the slow curl-up, with feet not held, is a better test of abdominal endurance. In the timed sit-up, the held feet, the raise to a sit-up position, and the emphasis on speed all tend to involve muscle groups other than the abdominals. The curl-up is preferred for both conditioning and testing.

Testing children's upper arm strength and endurance has been difficult. Pull-ups, in which one's entire body weight must be moved, simply can't be done by many children. Even if they increase their strength or endurance, they still may not be able to perform the pull-up and thus will score "0" in testing. Another activity sometimes used for upper arm testing, the flexed arm hang, is a static test and is more a test of pain tolerance than of muscular strength and endurance. The modified pull-up is a dynamic test that is suitable for all levels of strength. It also minimizes the effects of excess fat on the test score.

The one-mile run and skinfold measurement tests have concurrent validity in that they are highly correlated with the "gold standard" tests for cardiorespiratory endurance and relative leanness: maximal oxygen uptake and underwater weighing. All the test items have some construct validity in that the scores improve when people do appropriate physical conditioning and fall when they stop training.

Improvement of Test Accuracy

A test score includes the individual's *true score* plus *error*. The error can result from the testing environment, the equipment, the tester, or changes in the person being tested. Testers can take the following three actions to obtain more accurate results:

- Prepare the person to be tested.
- Organize the testing session.
- Pay attention to detail.

Prepare the Person to Be Tested

The best test results are found when people are prepared for testing—that is, when they have been told what test procedures will be used, have complied with pretest instructions, and are physically and mentally prepared to take the test. Figure 2.1 is a checklist that can be used to determine if an individual is ready to be tested.

The person to be tested

_____ 1.   understands test procedures.

_____ 2.   has practiced the test and is comfortable with it.

_____ 3.   understands starting and stopping procedures.

_____ 4.   has complied with all pretest instructions.

_____ 5.   is not ill or injured.

_____ 6.   has had proper warm-up.

Figure 2.1. Checklist for preparing person for testing.

Organize the Testing Session

Preparing the person for testing is only part of the test session organization. Equipment and personnel also must be ready if testing is to be accurate and efficient. Figure 2.2

is a checklist that can be used for organizing the entire session.

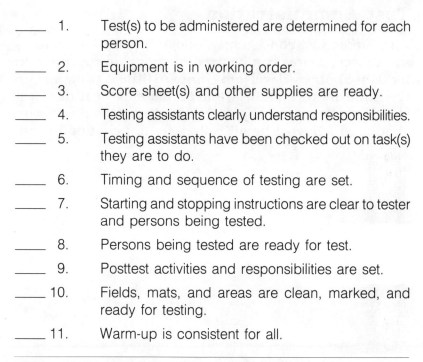

_____ 1.   Test(s) to be administered are determined for each person.

_____ 2.   Equipment is in working order.

_____ 3.   Score sheet(s) and other supplies are ready.

_____ 4.   Testing assistants clearly understand responsibilities.

_____ 5.   Testing assistants have been checked out on task(s) they are to do.

_____ 6.   Timing and sequence of testing are set.

_____ 7.   Starting and stopping instructions are clear to tester and persons being tested.

_____ 8.   Persons being tested are ready for test.

_____ 9.   Posttest activities and responsibilities are set.

_____ 10.   Fields, mats, and areas are clean, marked, and ready for testing.

_____ 11.   Warm-up is consistent for all.

Figure 2.2.   Checklist for testing session preparation.

Pay Attention to Detail

The one thing that most improves the accuracy of testing is attention to detail. Each tester must take care to prepare the person being tested, organize the testing session, and take data precisely if the results are to be accurate.

The YMCA recommends that a Y Fitness Specialist train those who will administer the test. The Specialist also may want to be involved in the test administration, especially of the skinfold measurements which require practice for accuracy.

Test Administration

All testers must consistently follow the same procedures so that test scores can be used to show improvement in individual fitness levels, to compare fitness programs in the same or other YMCAs, and to relate to the fitness test standards listed in chapter 3. The directions given here should be followed by all testers, both new and experienced ones.

ONE-MILE RUN

Equipment and personnel needed:

- Person to start and time runners
- Running space (if outdoors, look for holes and dips in path)
- Cones to mark the course (if needed)
- Area for warm-up
- 2 stopwatches (1 as a spare)
- 1 score sheet (see Figure 2.3) for each child
- Scratch paper for each child
- Pencils for half the children

Some days ahead of time, explain the purpose of the test. Tell the children that it determines how fast they can run a mile, which reflects the endurance of their heart and cardiovascular system.

Several times prior to the testing day, have the children practice running at a set submaximal pace, starting with one lap, then progressing to two, three, and so on. Table 2.2 provides lap times for practice. Help each child choose and practice a pace that can be continued for the entire mile. Do *not* administer the test until the children have had several practice sessions.

On the day of the test, select a level area (and mark it off if necessary) for the run. Figure 2.4 shows four possible course configurations.

When children run, they will need to have partners (for younger children, the partner may need to be an older child). The partner counts laps, telling the runner at the end of each lap how many laps are left, and records the runner's time on the score sheet.

Name _____   Birthdate _____

Girl   Boy   (circle one)

| | Date of test | | | |
Test item	Test 1 (Date)	Test 2 (Date)	Test 3 (Date)	Test 4 (Date)
One-mile run (min:sec)				
Triceps skinfold (mm)				
Calf skinfold (mm)				
Sum of triceps and calf skinfolds (mm)				
Percent fat (%)				

Modified curl-up (#)

Sit-and-reach test (in.)

Modified pull-ups (#)

Figure 2.3. Sample score sheet.

Table 2.2   Lap Times for Practicing for the One-Mile Run

Laps per mile	Age (years)					
			12-15		16 and over	
	6-8	9-11	Boys	Girls	Boys	Girls
4	2:00-4:00	1:40-3:40	1:30-3:30	1:50-3:50	1:20-3:00	1:40-3:40
8	1:00-2:00	0:50-1:50	0:45-1:45	0:55-1:55	0:40-1:30	0:50-1:50
16	0:30-1:00	0:25-0:55	0:23-0:53	0:28-0:58	0:20-0:45	0:25-0:55

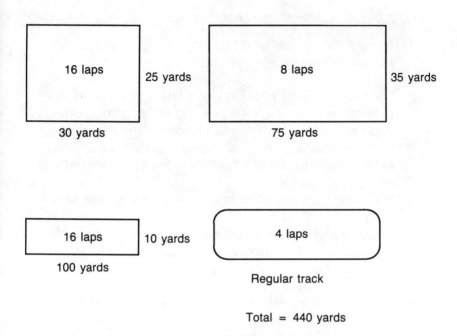

16 laps   25 yards

30 yards

8 laps   35 yards

75 yards

16 laps   10 yards

100 yards

4 laps

Regular track

Total = 440 yards

Figure 2.4.   Examples of one-mile run courses. *Note.* Adapted from *Health Related Physical Fitness Test Manual* (p. 10) by American Alliance for Health, Physical Education, Recreation and Dance, 1980, Reston, VA: Author. Reprinted by permission of the American Alliance for Health, Physical Education, Recreation and Dance, 1900 Association Drive, Reston, VA 22091.

For testing, follow these instructions:

1. Have children warm up by stretching, walking, and jogging slowly.
2. Pair them off.
3. Line up several children to run, and explain the procedure. They are to run the mile in the fastest time possible. Walking is allowed, but the goal is to cover the distance as quickly as they can. They are to listen for their finish times, which are called out by the timer.
4. Have the timer say "Ready, go!" and start the stopwatch.
5. While the children run, have the partners count the laps, telling the runners after each lap how many are left. The partners can use scratch paper and pencil to keep track of laps.
6. Have the timer call out the minutes and seconds as each child finishes.
7. Have each partner record the time to the nearest second on the score sheet. Runners should listen for their times as a back-up if the partners don't hear.
8. Tell runners to continue to walk for one lap after finishing to cool down.

TRICEPS AND CALF
SKINFOLD MEASUREMENT

Equipment and personnel needed:

- Trained test administrator (preferably a YMCA Fitness Specialist)
- Area where testing can be conducted privately
- 1 set of skinfold calipers (Harpenden, Lange, Fat-O-Meter, SlimGuide, or other)
- 1 score sheet for each child
- A pencil

Explain the purpose of the test to the children. Tell them the test determines the amount of fat they have in relation to their total body weight. Also tell them that the skinfold measurements will be taken in a private area where the score will not be shared with others.

The measurement sites are shown in Figure 2.5. The triceps skinfold is taken in the middle of the back of the arm, halfway between shoulder and elbow. The calf skinfold is taken on the *inside* of the calf at the point of the largest muscle mass (greatest circumference), with the child's foot on the bench and the knee slightly bent. When measuring, remember the following points:

- Always use the *right* side.
- Use a *vertical* fold for both sites.

For testing, see Figure 2.6 and follow these instructions:

1. Grasp between the thumb and forefinger the smallest amount of skin that will make a fold.
2. Lift the skinfold firmly and hold. Do *not* let go when measuring with the calipers.
3. Place the jaws of the calipers 1/2 inch above or below the fingers.
4. Slowly engage the calipers to measure the fold.
5. When the needle stops or the calipers have been taken to the designated point, read the skinfold to the nearest 0.5 millimeter.

6. Remove the calipers prior to letting go with the fingers.
7. Repeat the measurement 3 times. If all measurements are within 1 to 2 millimeters, take the middle score. If the difference between any two measurements is greater than 2 millimeters, repeat the procedure.

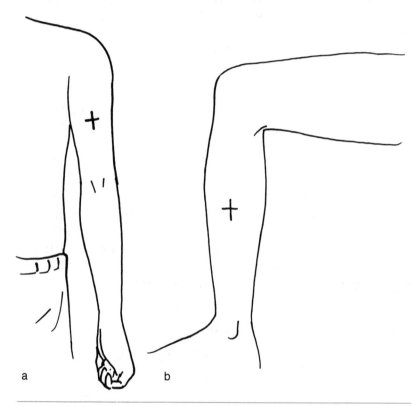

Figure 2.5.   Skinfold measurement sites: (a) tricep; (b) calf.

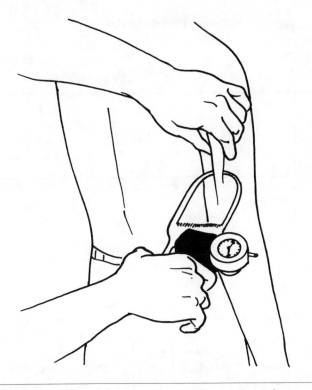

Figure 2.6. Skinfold measurement procedure.

To score, follow these instructions:

1. Record the number of millimeters for each site on the score sheet.
2. Add the two measurements and record the sum on the score sheet.
3. Use the chart in Figure 2.7 to determine the child's percent of body fat.
4. Record the percentage on the score sheet.

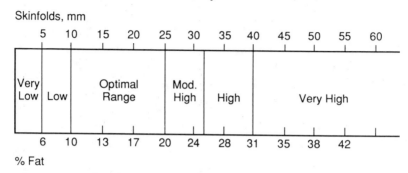

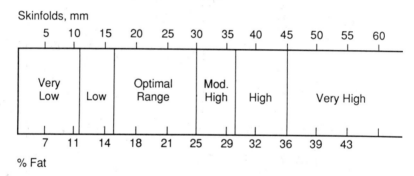

Figure 2.7. Chart for conversion of skinfold measurements to body fat percentages. *Note.* From "The Use of Skinfolds to estimate Body Fatness in Children and Youth" by T. G. Lohman, 1987, *Journal of Physical Education, Recreation & Dance*, **58**(9), p. 100. Reprinted by permission of the American Alliance for Health, Physical Education, Recreation and Dance, 1900 Association Drive, Reston VA 22091.

CURL-UPS

Equipment and personnel needed:

- A flat, padded surface
- 1 score sheet for each child
- A pencil

Explain the purpose of the test to the children. Tell them that the test determines the strength and endurance of their abdominal muscles, which help prevent low back problems.

Children will need partners to do curl-ups. The partner cups his or her hands beneath the child's head as the child exercises and counts the number of curl-ups done. Several children can be tested at the same time.

For testing, see Figure 2.8 and follow these instructions:

1. Pair children off.
2. Have the child being tested lie on his or her back with knees at about a 150° angle and arms extended, with fingers resting on the legs and pointing toward the knees. (Note: At the 150° angle, the knees are close to the floor.) *Do not hold or anchor the child's feet.*
3. Ask the child's partner to get behind the child with hands cupped under the child's head and to count the number of curl-ups performed.
4. Have the child curl up slowly until the fingertips touch the knees, then curl back down, doing about one curl every 3 seconds. The initial phase of the curl-up involves a flattening of the lower back (pelvic tilt), followed by a *slow* curling up of the upper spine, with hands sliding along the thighs until fingertips touch knees. The heels must remain in contact with the floor at all times. The child should return to the starting position by touching the partner's hands with the back of the head.

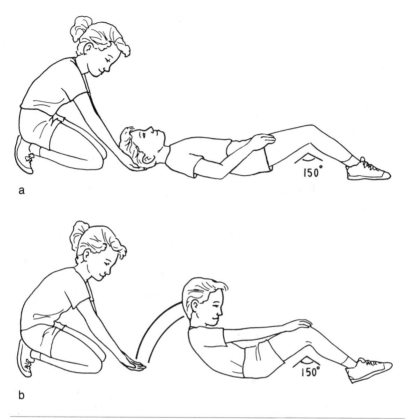

a

b

Figure 2.8.   Curl-ups: (a) down position; (b) up position. *Note.* Adapted from drawings from *Revised Canada Fitness Award Manual* (p. 11). Developed and distributed by Fitness and Amateur Sport Canada, Government of Canada, 1985, Ottawa, ON: Minister of Supply and Services, Canada. Copyright 1985 by Minister of Supply and Services, Canada.

5. Let the child do as many curl-ups as can be done without stopping, up to 40. *Stop* the test if the child (a) appears to have severe discomfort or pain; (b) is unable to maintain correct rhythm (stop after 3 times); or (c) displays poor technique, such as lifting the heels, throwing the hands forward, failing to touch the knees, not returning the head to the partner's hands, or failing to keep the knees at the correct angle (stop after 3 corrections).
6. When the child is finished, record on the score sheet the number of curl-ups performed.

SIT-AND-REACH TEST

Equipment and personnel needed:

- Area for warm-up
- Sit-and-reach box (see Figure 2.9 for specifications on how to build)
- 1 score sheet for each child
- A pencil

Explain the purpose of the test to the children. Tell them that it measures the flexibility of the low back and the back of the legs, which helps prevent low back problems.

Children should warm up prior to this test with the two static stretches shown in Figure 2.10. Each stretch should be done twice on each leg and held for 20 to 30 seconds.

For testing, see Figure 2.11 and follow these instructions:

1. Have the child take off his or her shoes and sit with feet shoulder-width apart and flat against the box.
2. Have the child place one hand on top of the other and extend the arms forward.
3. Keep the child's knees from bending by applying slight pressure to the child's upper legs.
4. Ask the child to reach forward *slowly* as far as possible 4 times. Tell the child not to lunge or rock forward, and to hold the fourth reach for at least 1 second.
5. Read the point that the longest finger on both hands reached while the fourth reach is being held.
6. Record on the score sheet the distance to the nearest 1/2 inch.

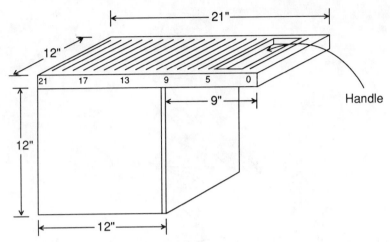

1. Using any sturdy wood or comparable construction material (3/4" plywood seems to work well), cut the following pieces.
   4 pieces—12" × 12"
   1 piece—12" × 21"
2. Assemble the pieces using nails or screws and wood glue.
3. Inscribe the top panel with 1/2" gradations. It is crucial that the 9" line be exactly in line with the vertical panel against which the child's feet are placed.
4. For carrying convenience, make a handle by cutting a 1" × 3" hole in the top panel.
5. Cover the apparatus with two coats of polyurethane sealer or shellac.
6. The measuring scale should extend from 0" at the handle end to 21" at the far end.

As an alternative to the sit-and-reach box, a yardstick can be affixed to the top of a bench. If this alternative is used, make sure to mount the yardstick so the 9" mark is in line with the vertical panel against which the child's feet are placed.

Figure 2.9.   Sit-and-reach box specifications. *Note.* From *Health Related Physical Fitness Test Manual* (p. 68) by American Alliance for Health, Physical Education, Recreation and Dance, 1980, Reston, VA: Author. Adapted by permission of the American Alliance for Health, Physical Education, Recreation and Dance, 1900 Association Drive, Reston VA 22091.

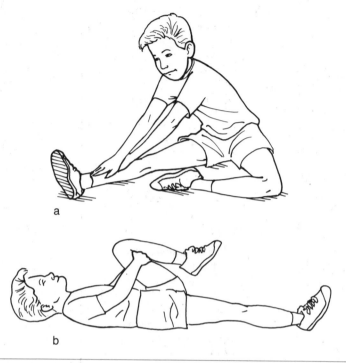

a

b

Figure 2.10. Warm-up stretches for sit-and-reach test: (a) modified hurdler's stretch; (b) knee to chest.

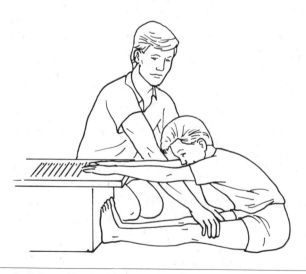

Figure 2.11. Sit-and-reach test.

MODIFIED PULL-UPS

Equipment and personnel needed:

- A pull-up box with bar and rubber bands (single or chained bands) (see Figure 2.12 for specifications on how to build)
- 1 score sheet for each child
- A pencil

Explain the purpose of the test to the children. Tell them that the test measures the muscular strength and endurance of their arms.

Before beginning testing, have the child being tested lie on his or her back with the head under the bar and shoulders between the uprights. Ask the child to reach straight up as high as possible with fingers extended toward the bar, while keeping the head and shoulders flat on the floor. Then place the bar through the drilled holes in the slot 1 to 1-1/2 inches beyond the child's extended fingers, and stretch the rubber band (or chain of rubber bands) across the pegs four down from the bar. (The pegs should be at the back of the stand, facing away from the child's feet.)

For testing, see Figure 2.13 and follow these instructions:

1. Have the child place hands on the bar using an overhand grip (palms facing out), with thumbs around the bar and arms in front of the rubber band.
2. Ask the child to pull up with the body fully extended (buttocks off the floor, legs straight with feet together and only heels touching the floor) until the chin touches the rubber band. The child should then lower the body until the arms are fully extended. Only the arms should be used in the pull-up, and they must be fully extended upon return to the starting position. No part of the body other than the heels may touch the floor, and the trunk and legs must remain straight throughout the test.

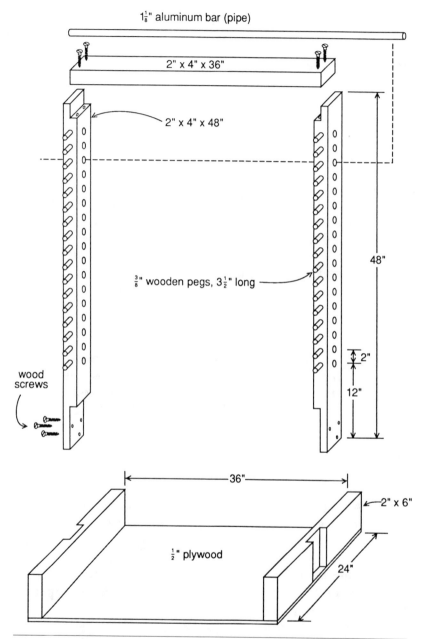

Figure 2.12. Assembly instructions for modified pull-up apparatus.

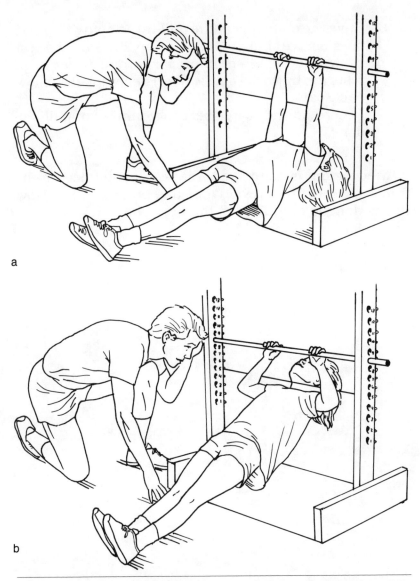

Figure 2.13. Modified pull-up: (a) down position; (b) up position. *Note.* Drawings based on photos from "The Modified Pull-Up Test" by R.R. Pate, J.G. Ross, T.A. Baumgartner, and R.E. Sparks, 1987, *Journal of Physical Education, Recreation & Dance,* **58**(9), p. 72. Reprinted by permission of the American Alliance for Health, Physical Education, Recreation and Dance, 1900 Association Drive, Reston, VA 22091.

3. Have the child repeat the pull-up as many times as possible without stopping, up to 20. *Stop* the test if the child exhibits improper form 3 times (e.g., rests the buttocks on the floor) or complains of low back pain.
4. Record on the score sheet the number of pull-ups done.

After testing is completed, the test results need to be translated into fitness evaluation and programming. How this is done is described in the next chapter.

CHAPTER 3

Application of Test Results to Fitness Programming

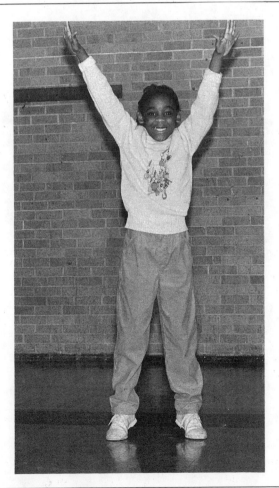

Testing is only one part of a physical fitness program. Just as important is the way that test scores are interpreted to participants and how that interpretation determines program activities. The YMCA Youth Fitness Test is meant to help children understand what the important components of fitness are and evaluate their own health status and fitness improvement over time.

The major thrust of any fitness program should be to promote fitness behaviors. While people may be interested in how their scores compare to others or to some standard, the goal of the fitness program should be to encourage them to be active in a variety of ways and to practice better health habits.

To achieve this goal, test scores can be used as a yardstick for improvement and for basic health. Standards for all test scores are included later in the chapter for this purpose. The standards are based on the information now available about health needs for children of all ages. They provide guidelines for feedback, but they should not be overemphasized.

Recognition of Fitness Gains

One incentive for children's participation in fitness programming is recognition, and test scores can help program leaders provide it. Recognition should be given for meeting any one of three criteria: Exhibiting fitness behaviors, reaching health-based test standards, and improving test scores.

Exhibiting Fitness Behaviors

Fitness behaviors such as exercising, following a nutritious diet, resting, avoiding substance abuse, and coping with stress are directly related to fitness test scores. The program leader should emphasize that these fitness behaviors are more essential than particular scores. It is more important for children to begin and continue regular physical activity than to score a certain time on an endurance run; and it is more important for children to eat a nutritious diet than to have a certain percentage of body fat. By emphasizing fitness behaviors, the program leader recognizes children for their efforts, which in the long run is the best way to improve fitness test scores. Overemphasis on test scores can discourage some participants.

Giving awards for specific fitness behaviors is recommended. Behaviors that might be rewarded include the following:

- Completion of a unit in the YMCA youth fitness program with at least 75% attendance
- Completion of two sports classes, such as swimming and soccer
- Running 10 miles a week for 10 weeks

Reaching Health-Based Test Standards

A common approach to test interpretation is to compare the person tested with others of the same gender and age. For instance, a test may show that a child ran faster on the one-mile run than 60% of children of the same sex and age. But although children or parents may ask for this type of feedback, it is probably the least useful in assessing a child's fitness. This kind of comparison may reflect a child's heredity and early experience more than a child's health. For some children, there may be limits to how much change can be achieved even with a lot of effort. Thus, the emphasis in a fitness program should not be on identifying who can run the fastest, but rather on helping *all* children to understand and to try to obtain or maintain healthy levels of all fitness components.

The feedback given after the first testing session should be based on whether the children meet health standards, not what percentage of the population they can "beat" on a test. That is why the test standards set for the YMCA Youth Fitness Test are based on what is needed for good health. For example, the percent fat given as a standard for young women is between 15% and 25% of total body weight (children and young men should have between 10% and 20%). It doesn't matter what percentage of the population currently is in that range. What does matter is that if people have less fat than the lower end of that range, they have health risks associated with having too little fat. If they have more fat than the upper end of the range, then their risk of developing (or worsening) major health problems increases.

The program leader should encourage all participants to try to reach and maintain the health standards for all fitness components. Health standards for children ages 6 to 17 appear in Tables 3.1, 3.2, and 3.3. Note that more research is needed to refine these standards, so they may have to be modified as more is discovered about the relationship between the test scores and positive health.

The health standards for boys and girls are the same through age 11; after that age there are separate standards. This differentiation is due to the fact that girls develop additional essential fat at puberty. The extra fat affects skinfold measurement and running times. Scores of girls older than 11 who have not reached puberty should be compared with standards for 11-year-olds. Breast development is probably the clearest indicator of additional essential fat and should determine whether a girl older than 11 is prepubescent or pubescent. There are no guidelines for this determination; it is a judgment to be made by the tester.

The fitness standards are grouped into three classifications: *good, borderline*, and *needs work*. Those whose scores fall into the *good* classification should be given an award and encouraged to maintain that level of fitness. Those with *borderline* scores should be helped to make minor modifications in their fitness habits to improve the specific fitness components on which they scored low. For example, a child who scores *borderline* on the 1-mile run should try to take part in more aerobic activities; if the

Table 3.1   Fitness Test Standards for Children Ages 6 to 11

Test item	Age (years)					
	6	7	8	9	10	11
One-mile run (min:sec)						
Good	15	14	13	12	11	10
Borderline	16-17	15-16	14-15	13-14	12-13	11-12
Needs work	≥18	≥17	≥16	≥15	≥14	≥13
Triceps and calf skinfolds (mm)						
Good	10-25	10-25	10-25	10-25	10-25	10-25
Borderline	27-30	27-30	27-30	27-30	27-30	27-30
Needs work	<5	<5	<5	<5	<5	<5
	>32	>32	>32	>32	>32	>32
Curl-ups						
Good	≥15	≥15	≥20	≥20	≥25	≥25
Borderline	8-12	8-12	10-15	10-15	15-20	15-20
Needs work	≤5	≤5	≤8	≤8	≤10	≤10

Sit-and-reach test (in.)						
Good	10	10	10	10	10	10
Borderline	6-8	6-8	6-8	6-8	6-8	6-8
Needs work	≤4	≤4	≤4	≤4	≤4	≤4
Modified pull-ups						
Good	≥5	≥6	≥7	≥8	≥9	≥10
Borderline	2-4	2-4	3-5	4-6	5-7	5-8
Needs work	≤1	≤1	≤2	≤2	≤3	≤3

Table 3.2   Fitness Test Standards for Girls Ages 12 to 17

Test item	Age (years)					
	12	13	14	15	16	17
One-mile run (min:sec)						
Good	12	12	11:30	11:30	11	11
Borderline	13-14	13-14	12:30-14	12:30-14	12-13	12-13
Needs work	⩾15	⩾15	⩾14:30	⩾14:30	⩾14	⩾14
Triceps and calf skinfolds (mm)						
Good	17-32	17-32	17-32	17-32	17-32	17-32
Borderline	34-38	34-38	34-38	34-38	34-38	34-38
Needs work	<15	<15	<15	<15	<15	<15
	>40	>40	>40	>40	>40	>40
Curl-ups						
Good	⩾25	⩾30	⩾30	⩾35	⩾35	⩾35
Borderline	15-20	17-25	17-25	20-30	20-30	20-30
Needs work	⩽10	⩽13	⩽13	⩽15	⩽15	⩽15

Sit-and-reach test (in.)						
Good	10	10	10	10	10	10
Borderline	6-8	6-8	6-8	6-8	6-8	6-8
Needs work	≤4	≤4	≤4	≤4	≤4	≤4
Modified pull-ups						
Good	≥7	≥8	≥9	≥10	≥10	≥10
Borderline	3-5	4-6	5-7	5-8	5-8	5-8
Needs work	≤2	≤2	≤3	≤3	≤3	≤3

Note. Use the norms for 11-year-old children for test scores of prepubescent girls.

Table 3.3   Fitness Test Standards for Boys Ages 12 to 17

Test item	Age (years)					
	12	13	14	15	16	17
One-mile run (min:sec)						
Good	10	9	9	8:30	8:30	8:30
Borderline	11-12	10-11	10-11	9:30-11	9:30-11	9:30-11
Needs work	≥13	≥12	≥12	≥11:30	≥11:30	≥11:30
Triceps and calf skinfolds (mm)						
Good	10-25	10-25	10-25	10-25	10-25	10-25
Borderline	27-30	27-30	27-30	27-30	27-30	27-30
Needs work	<5	<5	<5	<5	<5	<5
	>32	>32	>32	>32	>32	>32
Curl-ups						
Good	≥25	≥30	≥30	≥35	≥35	≥35
Borderline	15-20	17-25	17-25	20-30	20-30	20-30
Needs work	≤10	≤12	≤12	≤15	≤15	≤15

Sit-and-reach test (in.)						
Good	10	10	10	10	10	10
Borderline	6-8	6-8	6-8	6-8	6-8	6-8
Needs work	≤4	≤4	≤4	≤4	≤4	≤4
Modified pull-ups						
Good	≥11	≥12	≥13	≥15	≥15	≥15
Borderline	6-9	6-10	7-11	9-13	9-13	9-13
Needs work	≤4	≤4	≤5	≤7	≤7	≤7

score is low on the sit-and-reach test, the child should do more midtrunk stretching during warm-up and cool-down. Children with scores in the *needs work* area need special attention. They will not be able to achieve the fitness standards quickly, and they may not know how to improve their scores. With help from the program leader, they can learn what activities to increase (perhaps doing the activities with a program leader or a partner initially) and set some realistic goals for improving toward the fitness standard.

Improving Scores

The most important question for a fitness participant is not what his or her health is like at this moment, but rather what it will be like in 6 months, 2 years, or 20 years! After the child knows how he or she compares with health-based standards, the next step is to develop reasonable goals for the period before the next test. This is especially true for those children who score in the bottom region of the fitness test. The program leader should work with each child to develop goals and should provide the best activity recommendations possible based on fitness knowledge (type of exercise, total work, intensity, frequency, etc.) and the child's interests. Awards should be presented for achievement of individual goals.

If a child is very unfit, the program leader may want to set subgoals with the child. It would be discouraging to a child to discuss one-mile run standards if he or she could only walk a quarter of a mile without stopping. The initial goal for that child may be to work up to walking a mile without stopping. In another case, a child who has a lot of fat may aim at decreasing calories and increasing exercise to lose 1 pound of weight every 2 weeks. This subgoal might lead to the broader fitness goal of losing 6 pounds over the next 3 months.

In some cases the health standards given in Tables 3.1 through 3.3 may not be appropriate or reasonable, and individual goals should be established. For example, the one-mile run standards cannot be used for someone who works out by swimming or is in a wheelchair.

In summary, when fitness test scores are interpreted to children and parents, the program leader needs to keep three things in mind:

- Emphasize health status rather than comparison with others.
- Emphasize potential for improvement rather than current status.
- Provide activity recommendations for each child based on test data and the child's preferences.

Awards should be provided for all children who demonstrate fitness behaviors, who meet fitness standards, or who reach individual fitness improvement goals.

Program Development

Analysis of test scores and other data from different fitness classes can help program leaders decide how classes can be improved. For instance, questions such as the following can be asked:

- How many children drop out of various classes?
- How much improvement is being made in cardiorespiratory endurance, relative leanness, muscular strength and endurance, and low back strength and flexibility?
- How many injuries occur in certain types of classes?

Answers to these questions can help leaders improve the fitness activities they offer.

Another use of test scores is to help educate the public about children's fitness programs at the Y and to get positive attention for them. Statistics about how many participants make large fitness gains, the total amount of fat lost by participants in a year, or the number of miles participants have run during the year can be impressive promotional tools. Careful testing, record keeping, and analysis can provide helpful information about Y programs to the public.

The tests described in this booklet can be used in conjunction with the new YMCA youth fitness program lesson plans (Thomas et al., in press). While this booklet describes how the fitness components can be measured and evaluated, the youth fitness program lesson plans describe specific fitness activities for children of all ages.

References

□

American Alliance for Health, Physical Education, Recreation and Dance. (1980). *Health related physical fitness test manual*. Reston, VA: Author.

American Alliance for Health, Physical Education, Recreation and Dance. (1988). *Physical best*. Reston, VA: Author.

American College of Sports Medicine. (1988). Opinion statement on physical fitness in children and youth. *Medicine and Science in Sports and Exercise*, **20**(4), 422-423.

American Heart Association. (1986). Coronary risk factor modification in children: Exercise. *Circulation*, **74**(2), 1189A-1191A.

Franks, B.D., & Howley, E.T. (1989). *Fitness leader's handbook*. Champaign, IL: Human Kinetics.

Government of Canada. (1985). *Canada fitness award*. Ottawa, ON: Minister of Supply and Services, Canada.

Howley, E.T., & Franks, B.D. (1986). *Health/fitness instructor's handbook*. Champaign, IL: Human Kinetics.

Lohman, T.G. (1987). The use of skinfolds to estimate body fatness in children and youth. *Journal of Physical Education, Recreation & Dance*, **58**(9), 98-102.

Pate, R.R., Ross, J.G., Baumgartner, T.A., & Sparks, R.E. (1987). The modified pull-up test. *Journal of Physical Education, Recreation & Dance*, **58**(9), 71-73.

Thomas, K., Lee, A., & Thomas, J. (in press). *YMCA youth fitness program*. Champaign, IL: Human Kinetics.

Resources

American Alliance for Health, Physical Education, Recreation and Dance. (1984). *Technical manual: Health related physical fitness*. Reston, VA: Author.

American College of Sports Medicine. (1985). *Guidelines for graded exercise testing and exercise prescription* (3rd ed.). Philadelphia: Lea & Febiger.

Anderson, B. (1980). *Stretching*. Bolinas, CA: Shelter Publications.

Blair, S.N., Jacobs, D.R., & Powell, K.E. (1985). Relationships between exercise or physical activity and other health behaviors. *Public Health Reports,* **100**, 180-188.

Blair, S.N., Painter, P., Pate, R.R., Smith, L.K., & Taylor, C.B. (Eds.) (1988). *Resource manual for exercise testing and prescription*. Philadelphia: Lea & Febiger.

Bubb, W.J. (1986). Relative leanness. In E.T. Howley & B.D. Franks, *Health/fitness instructor's handbook* (pp. 51-79). Champaign, IL: Human Kinetics.

Corbin, C.B. (1987). Physical fitness in the K-12 curriculum: Some defensible solutions to perennial problems. *Journal of Physical Education, Recreation & Dance,* **58**(7), 49-54.

Corbin, C.B., and Lindsey, R. (1988). *Concepts of physical fitness* (6th ed.). Dubuque, IA: W.C. Brown.

Cureton, T.K. (1965). *Physical fitness and dynamic health*. New York: Dial Press.

Dotson, C. (1988). Health fitness standards: Aerobic endurance. *Journal of Physical Education, Recreation & Dance,* **59**(7), 26-31.

Fit Youth Today. (1986). *Fit Youth Today program manual*. Austin, TX: American Health and Fitness Foundation.

Fox, K.R., & Biddle, S.J.H. (1988). The use of fitness tests. *Journal of Physical Education, Recreation & Dance,* **59**(2), 47-53.

Franks, B.D., Morrow, J.R., & Plowman, S.A. (1989). Youth fitness testing: Politics, validation, and planning. *Quest*, **40**(2), 187-199.

Gober, B.E., & Franks B.D. (1988). The physical and fitness education of young children. *Journal of Physical Education, Recreation & Dance*, **59**(7), 57-61.

Going, S. (1988). Physical best: Body composition in the assessment of youth fitness. *Journal of Physical Education, Recreation & Dance*, **59**(7), 32-36.

Golding, L.A., Myers, C.R., & Sinning, W.E. (Eds.) (1989). *Y's way to physical fitness* (3rd ed.). Champaign, IL: Human Kinetics.

Institute for Aerobics Research. (1988). *Fitnessgram*. Dallas: Author.

Jackson, A.S., & Pollock, M.L. (1985). Practical assessment of body composition. *The Physician and Sportsmedicine*, **13**(5), 76-90.

Katch, F.I., & McArdle, W.D. (1977). *Nutrition, weight control, and exercise*. Boston: Houghton Mifflin.

Kraus, H., & Raab, W. (1961). *Hypokinetic disease*. Springfield, IL: Charles C Thomas.

Liemohn, W.P. (1988). Flexibility and muscular strength. *Journal of Physical Education, Recreation & Dance*, **59**(7), 37-40.

Melleby, A. (1982). *The Y's way to a healthy back*. Piscataway, NJ: New Century.

Pollock, M.L., Wilmore, J.H., & Fox, S.M. (1984). *Exercise in health and disease*. Philadelphia: W.B. Saunders.

Seefeldt, V., & Vogel, P. (1986). *The value of physical activity*. Reston, VA: American Alliance for Health, Physical Education, Recreation and Dance.

Sharkey, B.J., (1984). *Physiology of fitness*. Champaign, IL: Human Kinetics.

Sharpe, G.S., & Liemohn, W.P. (1986). Strength, endurance, and flexibility. In E.T. Howley & B.D. Franks, *Health/fitness instructor's handbook* (pp. 99-113). Champaign: IL: Human Kinetics.

Sharpe, G.S., Liemohn, W.P., & Snodgrass, L.B. (1988). Exercise prescription and the low back—Kinesiological factors. *Journal of Physical Education, Recreation & Dance*, **59**(9), 74-79.

U.S. Department of Health and Human Services. (1980). *Promoting health/preventing disease: Objectives for the nation.* Washington, DC: U.S. Government Printing Office.

U.S. Department of Health and Human Services. (1981). *Exercise and your heart.* Washington, DC: U.S. Government Printing Office.

Williams, P.C. (1974). *Low back and neck pain.* Springfield, IL: Charles C Thomas.

Williams, R.L., & Long, J.D. (1983). *Toward a self-managed life style.* Boston: Houghton Mifflin.

Wilmore, J.H. (1986). *Sensible fitness.* Champaign, IL: Human Kinetics.